38 Ways to Increase Testosterone Naturally.

INDEX OF CONTENTS

22- Do not eat this.
23- Soya.
24. Water is the most important thing.
25- Do strength training.
26- HIIT Training.
27- Move!
28- Run.
29- Calistenia.
30- Never overtrain.
31- Multivitamin Supplements.
Ashwaghanda will help you a lot.
33- Probiotics.
34- Less estrogens!
35- The Tongkat Ali.
36- Ginger increases testosterone.
37- Goat herb in heat.
38- Mucuna Pruriens.

I've been a long time studying what I call the success hormone, testosterone is not just an indicator in your analysis, such as triglycerides, glucose, etc, I have the firm condition that is much more important, even more important, around testosterone is where a man's personality is forged: his actions, success with women, business, relationships, etc, all that are greatly affected by testosterone levels....

Everything you see here is backed by personal experience or / and scientific studies, but no matter how good or bad this guide is you have to take into account that increasing your testosterone levels does not correspond to me, if not to you, the responsibility to improve your health in the last stay is yours and yours alone, is not mine, not even your doctor's, if you continue reading this book and apply his advice you have to record this on fire, you should also have not only this guide as a reference, many other guides, nutritionist, of course to your doctor, each case is personal and unique. The above takes responsibility for your health and life.

There are many factors that influence testosterone levels: nutrition, supplementation, lifestyle, macronutrients, testicular health, sex, and a long and extensive etc.

Testosterone, what is it, how is it produced, effects, brief introduction etc.

How Testosterone Is Produced.

Testosterone is the male hormone par excellence, it is responsible for many of the characteristics associated with men: deep voice, greater muscle mass, aggressiveness, competitiveness, greater sexual desire, etc.

Testosterone is produced when the hypothalamus releases small waves of "gonadotropin-releasing hormone or simply GnRH, this gland moves to the pituitary gland, there is where the hormone GnRH stimulates the secretion of other hormones, which are follicle-stimulating hormone (or FSH) and luteinizing hormone (or LH), these are called gonadotropin hormones.

The gonadropin hormones (LH and FSH) will later go to the testicles through your spine, there FSH stimulates the creation of sperm, at the same time LH stimulates the testicular cells of leydig, these cells produce testosterone using cholesterol.

When testosterone has been manufactured, it is distributed through the blood. There the testosterone ends up in different parts or doing different processes, etc, are as follows:

–   Free Testosterone: part of this testosterone will remain free in your blood, bio available.

–   Androgen receptors: Another part will remain in the androgen receptors that are in your body.
–   Another binds to the albumin and SHBG becoming an inactive part of it.
–   Estrogen: Estrogen is also known as female hormone, a part of the available testosterone that is converted to estrogen.

This whole process can be influenced through nutrition, training, lifestyle and supplementation. All this is what we will cover in this guide... but... all of this really matters to you, it doesn't stop being really interesting but you're not here to get a science class, it's here to stop feeling so bad and increase your testosterone levels, more motivation, more muscle, more energy, more competitiveness, more sexual desire, more health, etc, etc, the number of advantages are innumerable and you can get this if you change your nutrition, your training, your lifestyle, supplementation, way of thinking, etc, these are the 38 ways to increase your testosterone naturally:

1- Sleep as much as you need.

Sleeping 4, 6 or 8 hours can significantly influence your testosterone levels.

A sleep restriction, even if "only" partial, can greatly affect your testosterone levels, a study in a laboratory concluded that restricting to 5 hours of sleep rest can lower your testosterone levels by up to 15%.

Another study carried out by Peneve stated that men who slept 4 hours approximately had testosterone levels of between 200

- 300 ng/dl on average, parallel to those who slept 8 hours (approximately) had levels of up to 700 ng/dl.

Another study done by "Gov" showed something very similar with 530 Chinese men, this study related greater hours of sleep with higher levels of testosterone both total and free, specifically each extra hour of sleep produced 15% more testosterone. You have all the links to the studies in the bibliography area at the end of the book.

2- Muscular mass and definition.

You can be very thin, it doesn't matter if you have big muscles or not, what you can't do is be fat, that's forbidden, you have to be defined. The body mass index should always be around 10 - 12% if you want to have high testosterone.

Generally speaking the higher the fat index in your body, the lower the testosterone levels. If you're fat it's likely that you have low testosterone.

Of course there is also a correlation between muscle mass and testosterone, more muscle equals more testosterone. If you lose weight and get strong you will look spectacular, you will also feel extremely good.

Fat people have lower testosterone levels, but why? If you have a lot of fat in your body you will also have a lot more aromatase enzyme activity which will cause more testosterone to turn into estrogen.

Obesity linked to low testosterone levels is quite linked to high oxidative stress, metabolic syndrome and low insulin sensitivity.

Remember that this is NOT something you are doomed to, you can always get to exercise and lose weight, and choose.

If you are below 8% body fat you are in the red zone, and this will affect your testosterone levels, why is that? It is because the trroid hormone substantially decreases its activity.

3- Relax and don't stress.

Stress is one of the worst things that can happen to you if you want to have testosterone levels, it's true that it's not easy, I understand.

Stress increases your levels of homone cortisol which is the main stress hormone, cortisol is a catabolic hormone that reduces your testosterone levels.

Obviously stress is good for something, do not try to reduce your cortisol levels to 0 because you will have a hard time and if you get it will be at the cost of your life.

Do what you consider to lower your levels of cortisol: change partners, find another job, leave your parents' house, change country (wars, economic crisis or not so extreme situations) Cortisol destroys muscle fiber and causes great oxidative damage to your body, also composed of the same material as testosterone (pregnenolone). If you have very high levels of cortisol you will have problems, because cortisol destroys the free testosterone that is inside the testicles and in your veins.

4- Endocrine disruptors and plastics are your enemies.

An endocrine disruptor is a substance or compound that disrupts your endocrine system (hormones, glands, receptors in the cell, etc.), this could affect your development and/or your reproduction.

These substances or compounds are normally found in plastics, preservatives, pesticides, personal care products, etc. The vast majority of chemicals to which we are exposed are harmless, but there is a small part of these chemicals that could influence your hormone production and other body functions.

Some of them are:

- **Parabetes**: they are usually preservatives that are in most cosmetics, usually starting with "methyl", "butyl", "ethyl", "propyl" and "heptyl-". They are in sun lotions, lubricants, hand creams, moisturizers, shaving gels, shampoos, toothpaste, food additives, and so on. Parabens are xenoestrogens and may have some affinity with your body's estrogen receptors.

- **BPA**, or better known as **bisfenoal A**, interacts similarly to the hormones in your body and is related to low levels of testosterone and erectile dysfunction. It is one of the most used substances in the world, is on the surface of plastics mostly, bisphenol is used to harden plastics and epoxy resin.

- **Phthalates** and low testosterone levels are interrelated, phthalates are similar to BPA in that they are in plastics, but instead of hardening the plastic they make it more flexible. They are also in personal care items such as stabilizers and/or emulsifying agents.

- **Benzophenones** are BP-1, BP-2, BP-3, etc. They are mainly used in sunscreens, although in general they can be found in many personal care items. Benzophenones are closely related to the reduction of enzymes needed to produce testosterone. It is used because it absorbs UV radiation from the sun and improves permeability.

- **Triclocarban and Triclosan.** They are in soaps, lotions, hand sanitizers and a long etc.. They reduce testicular production of testosterone. They are supposed to be antibacterial.

And how can you stop being exposed to this?, simple, stop using them, reduce their use to 0 or almost 0, how? Use non-plastic glass bottles, use natural products, don't eat canned food, etc. These are just one of the few things you can do to improve your testosterone levels.

5- Sex is important.

Not only is sex pleasurable, it also increases testoterone. Apparently the pheromones, dopamine, the feeling of power, etc. makes your testosterone levels are higher.

In one study it has been seen that men just by visiting an alternate club their testosterone levels increased up to 14% and this only with seeing and entering, those men who had sex had an increase of 70%.

6- Medications and their side effects.

The pharmaceutical industry exists for the money and the pharmaceutical companies aim to maximize the profits of their shareholders, these companies earn trillions of dollars each year. this is obvious but many forget when it comes to the truth.

Some drugs are important for people's health, but most treat the symptom not the origin, this is because they do not want people to be cured and the more sick the greater the amount of benefits.

If a natural product cannot be patented you will not be prescribed it, even if this is better than the drugs. They go all the way to the world to invent diseases.

Please keep in mind, your health is at stake. These are the drugs that lower your testosterone levels:

- **Many SSRIs (antidepressants)** are "famous" for lowering libido and also reducing testosterone levels.
- **Acid reducers such as:** Tagamet, Cidemetidine, etc.
- **Some beta-blockers and tranquilizers.**
- A medication for type 2 diabetes called **Sylfonylurea**.
- **Statins** and other drugs that interfere with cholesterol synthesis.
- **Medications for hair loss**, such as finasteride and dutasteride.
- A blood pressure drug called **Spironolactone**.
- **Some antifungal drugs**, such as ketoconazole
- **Corticosteroids.**
- **Analgesics based on opiates.**

Probably there are more, but we are still not aware of them or studies have not been done to prove it.

7. Your body posture.

Your body language plays a fundamental role in your hormones, it is scientifically proven that **having more dominant postures** (occupy more space, curved back, breast removal, etc.) results in an increase in testosterone, specifically an increase of 20%, on the other hand submissive postures (occupy less space, curved back, drooping shoulders, avoid eye contact, etc.) result in lower testosterone levels.

8- Money

Earning money gives happiness, **money today is equal to freedom**, with money you can buy many things including medical treatments to increase testosterone, supplements to improve your health and increase testosterone, etc, etc, but that is not the most important thing to have a lot of money will change your self-perception, **you will feel much better being who you are.**

Win something, win a tournament, win money, win any kind of competition is related to higher levels of testosterone. For example in a study on "brokers" observed an increase in testosterone levels of up to 78% when they earned a lot of money.

9- Your testicles.

Almost 100% of the testosterone you make in your body is made in the testicles, so if you have poor testicular health you will have problems with testosterone.
The testosterone in your testicles is made **specifically in the cells of leydig.**

Your testicles should always be a little colder than the rest of your body, what can you do about it?
- **Sleeping naked**

- Wear loose-fitting underwear.
- Take a cold shower.

There is a condition called **testicular varicocele** that consists of
 in which you have blocked or semi-blocked veins in your testicles or/and
you have veins that simply don't work properly in your testicles. Not
working properly does not reach the blood supply to the cells of leydig,
this makes your testicles produce much less testosterone, this is solved
with surgery. There are also people who say that they have experienced
improvements with massages.

10 - Alcohol

Alcohol is bad for testosterone and for your health in general, alcohol will
damage your health and lower your testosterone levels, I personally
believe that alcohol to be eliminated completely, some say that if you
only have a beer or a glass of wine from time to time nothing happens,
not true, affects, to a lesser extent but affects. Studies show that facts with
rodents resulted in a reduction of testicle by 50% after eating a diet where
5% of calories came from alcohol.

This has also been observed in men.
People who drink a lot, i.e. are alcoholics, usually have very low
testosterone levels and very high estrogen levels.

Obviously if you consume less alcohol your testosterone levels will be
less affected, for example 2 glasses of wine equals a 7% decrease in
testosterone levels.

My advice is not to deceive yourself, alcohol is a drug, it is bad for your
health, no matter how socially accepted it is, leave it.

11. Your Calorie Intake Matters.

In order to create enough testosterone your body requires a minimum of
calories. Calorie deficits are not good for your testosterone because your
body will pause your reproductive system, i.e. stop producing
testosterone in your testicles and use the energy for other more important
functions.

I'm not talking about extreme heat regimens like you can find in wars, postwar or third world countries. For example, a study showed that the group of men who consumed 1880 calories per day and had a correct diet and exercise had 30% less testosterone than another group of sedentary men who consumed 2841 calories.
Unless you're fat, you should be eating more calories.

12. You eat too much protein.

If you want to build muscle or produce testosterone you need protein, but in the world of fitness is preached with excess protein consumption. **An excess of protein will not only not help you increase your muscles** (since the muscles have a limit of absorption), it will also reduce your testosterone levels.
A high protein diet also increases levels of cortisol (stress hormone) which destroys testosterone.
The optimal amount of protein to boost your testosterone is 22-23%.

13. Carbohydrates And More Carbohydrates.

Carbohydrates have become the satan of nutrition, I've heard things like that people don't need carbohydrates or that obesity is a consequence of ingesting carbohydrates, which is not true, it's the excess calories that makes you fatten, no matter if they are fats, proteins, carbohydrates, sugar, breads, lettuces, etc, what matters is the number of calories, not the type of nutrients or foods. No man should undergo a low-carbohydrate diet as it reduces testosterone levels and increases cortisol.

Carbohydrate intake should be around 40%.

14. Fats.

I've seen serial killers with more popularity than fats. **Fats are very important** and perform various functions within your body: **creation of cell membranes, participation in the creation of testosterone, etc,** you need fats no matter what they say. Saturated and monounsaturated fats are very good if you want to increase your testosterone levels, while polyunsaturated fats and trans fats are bad for your testosterone.

15. Veganism is mostly bad.

I'm sorry to be the one to tell you but being vegetarian is not good, if you want to increase your testosterone levels you shouldn't have a vegan or vegetarian diet.

Vegan/vegetarian diets are often deficient in amino acids, cholesterol, and saturated fats, these three substances are key to producing adequate levels of testosterone.

Of course **there is also the possibility that you have a calorie deficit with this type of diet**, because of **vegetables tend to have fewer calories.** There are in fact several studies that state that this type of vegan/vegetarian diets increase the levels of SHBG which causes the levels of free testosterone to be reduced.

Of course there is a way to have high testosterone and have a vegan/vegetarian diet, but it would be hard, **if you take in enough calories, take in quality fats (nuts, olive oil and coconut) it is much more likely that you can have optimal testosterone levels while enjoying the benefits of a vegetarian diet (which are many).**

16. Ecological food.

In organic food and in normal food the nutrients are the same, a vitamin D is a vitamin D, an amino acid is an amino acid, etc, there is no doubt about that. **The only difference is that non-organic food has pesticides, herbicides, insecticides, etc,** these chemicals are usually poisonous.

Scientists analyzed almost 40 chemicals used as pesticides in agriculture, 30 of them were antiandrogens, ie negatively influence the production of male sex hormones.

Glyphosate, which is probably the most widely used herbicide in the world, negatively influences the production of testosterone, specifically "attacks" the cells of leydig (which is where testosterone is produced).

Farmers who work in fields where pesticides are used produce less sperm and sex hormones than those who worked on organic farms. This can be seen in virtually every study done with every agricultural chemical such as organophosphates, vinclozolin, PCBs and laatrazine.s.

What can you do?

- Eat organic food.
- Do not work in the agricultural industry.
- Do not live near fields.

17. Milk

Milk has many estrogen hormones, this is mainly to keep cows pregnant throughout the year. The hormone GnRH (or gonadotropin releasing hormone) is inhibited by the increase in estrogen and progesterone, all this leads to a drop in testosterone in men, the effects of milk on your testosterone can last up to 20 days.

Just don't drink milk.

18. Testosterone is made from CHOLESTEROL.

The body of a man of average size and weight creates 1.25 grams of cholesterol per day (0.002755778 pounds) and has 35 grams (approximately) in the cell membranes. There is a relationship between dietary cholesterol levels and testosterone levels, usually **the more cholesterol you consume, the better for your testosterone,** there are already studies that state that there is no relationship between the consumption of cholesterol and its presence in blood (at least in the long term) so you should not worry about the intake of it. Remember **even if you decide not to consume cholesterol, your body will still create it** in the liver, reproductive organs and adrenal glands.

Conclusion: **sex hormones are created using cholesterol, the more cholesterol consumed in the diet** and the more HDL cholesterol in your blood, the higher your testosterone levels will be. **Take the egg yolks** needed to maintain your testosterone levels.

19. The Coffee.

Coffee makes you produce more cortisol and adrenaline, as it stimulates the adrenal glands. Cortsisol destroys testosterone. All that extra energy you feel when you drink coffee is a product of cortisol and adrenaline, **is not good for your testosterone** so you should limit it or eliminate it tomally. The only use you could give to coffee would be as a stimulant before training, the intensity the training will be greater, burn more fat and your testosterone levels will be higher.

20. Fasting.

The bodybuilding industry preaches that you have to eat a lot and continuously for muscle growth and high levels of testosterone. The industry talks about 6 small meals throughout the day. The truth is that **the time between meals do not influence our metabolism.** If you eat less, the muscle is not destroyed, nor does it stop growing, etc. In fact after a short fast, androgen receptors are more receptive to testosterone, which is why **fasting can be beneficial if you want to increase your testosterone.** I personally do not recommend doing long fasts, if you do you should consult your doctor.

21. Eat more of this type of food.

If you want to increase your testosterone levels you should eat foods that:

- **Have plenty of micronutrients.**
- **Many antioxidants.**
- **Many saturated fats.**
- **Organic meat.**
- Etc.

If I tell you this, it's probably not very clear to you, so I've made a more detailed list:

- **Vegetables:** Avocados, potatoes, pomegranates, garlic, onions.
- **Meats:** Eggs, veal, oysters, organic bacon.
- **Spices:** Parsley, Ginger, Sodium Bicarbonate, Yogurt.
- **Nuts:** Raisins, cocoa seeds.
- **Fats and Oils:** Extra Virgin Olive Oil, Extra Virgin Coconut Oil.

22. Don't eat this.

In the same way that some foods can increase testosterone levels, others can reduce them, some are: **alcohol, green tea, mint, licorice, hierbabuenasoja vegetable oils and nuts with Polyunsaturated Fatty Acids.**

23. Soya.

High levels of estrogen are associated with low levels of testosterone, soy has Isoflavones (genistein, daidzein and glycitein) **that act as phytoestrogens,** these phytoestrogens are similar to estrogen and your body confuses these phytoestrogens are confused by your body by phytoesrogens, this makes your testosterone levels drop, this is at least what some studies say, others simply say there is no relationship between soy consumption and low levels of tesosterone. I rarely take soy because of studies that say it can affect testosterone levels and especially goitrogens that are compounds that affect the creation of thyroid hormones. Thyroids are very important if you want to have good health, motivation and high energy levels.

24. Water is the most important thing.

Water is the basis of life, you can go a long time without eating, without eating a good diet, not exercising, etc, but what happens if you go a long time without drinking water? You will die.

Water is very important, **the vast majority of people don't consume enough. More level dehydration increases cortisol levels, cortisol destroys testosterone.** If this happens during exercise, it's even worse.

25. Do strength training.

One of the consequences of strength training is that the receptivity of your androgen receptors in your muscles and testosterone levels increase. Testosterone increases in both the long and short term.

In addition **not only increases testosterone directly, thanks to strength training you will be more attractive and increase confidence in ourselves, this will increase your testosterone indirectly.**

Improvements in strength training are not only reduced to testosterone, muscle, etc, **it also improves the nervous system.**

But what's a strength training? **to train strength you have to: lift a lot of weight, do general exercises that use a lot of muscles, do short but very intense exercises.**

26. HIIT training.

HIIT training consists of exercising at very short intervals of very high intensity agreed with very short descending periods. The consequence of this type of training **is the activation of fast-contracting muscle fibers, increased testosterone, lactic acid, DHEA, growth hormone and DHT.**

If you start doing HIIT training you will notice a lot of benefits in all aspects of your life.

27. Move!

If you think that going to the gym a little and training a little is enough you are very wrong, we live in extremely sedentary societies and if you are in an office working most of the time you will notice how your health improves if you move a little. **You have to move! Do whatever it takes: walking, gardening, paintball, whatever, the point is to move.**

28. Running.

Long-term training such as a cyclist or marathon runner **can substantially reduce your testosterone, as well as increase cortisol.** Probably if you are doing marathons or similar you will find it difficult to leave because you may be addicted, but try to reduce it periodically, you can replace this type of training by strength training, HIIT, gym, swimming and so on. The exception here is swimming, which although it is a long-term training similar to running, does not lower your testosterone levels.

29. Calisthenics

Calisthenics consists of doing physical exercises with your own weight. This type of training **increases testosterone, as well as the receptivity of your androgen receptors.**

30. Never overtrain

Your body needs to rest, when you do physical exercise, especially if it is a workout where strength is required, you are breaking muscle fibers, these fibers need time to repair, if you train when your muscles are not ready you will be overtraining, you will not get the benefits of exercise, your testosterone will drop, etc, if you still want to train more and better, you should inform yourself and talk to your doctor to weigh the injections of substances like steroids, I personally would not make that decision, but if you are going to do it well with medical supervision, not by yourself.

If you do calisthenics, HITT or just go to the gym you will have to rest, you can not be every day training, because your body can not recover, **you can exercise a maximum of 5 days per week**, no more, the rest of the days you must rest and allow your body, your muscles, your hormonal system to recover for the next training sessions.

Remember also that **the training must always be progressive**, your exercise session must be more intense than today, but less intense than yesterday. This is a way to get out of your comfort zone, in a study with sedentary and normal people it was observed that you experienced higher levels of testosterone after training than professional athletes. These people were common people and trails, but thanks to the training they left their comfort zone and forced their body (and their hormones) to adapt, instead for professional athletes training was routine and not a challenge.

Conclusion: If you want to train more intensively every day to enjoy higher levels of testosterone you will have to devote some time to rest, **going to the gym when you're not recovered from the day before doesn't make sense and will affect your hormone levels.**

Do you like the book?

<u>CLICK HERE TO LEAVE ME YOUR OPINION ON AMAZON</u>

If you're not sure leave me a review later...

31. Multivitamin Supplements.

Many of us have micronutrient deficiencies (vitamin and / or minerals), this affects all levels of our lives, affects us professionally, in sex, love, etc. and of course health, specifically in terms of testosterone levels. **the most important minerals are magnesium, vitamin D and zinc,** of course there are many more and absolutely all affect to a greater or lesser extent, so I would recommend that you do this:

A) Eat a varied and abundant diet (unless you are fat).
B) Drink plenty of fruit.

C) Himalaya´s Salt, this is the one I take.
D) Drink shakes of vegetables each week (not fruit).

Es muy dificil, si no imposible tomar todos los micronutrientes solo con la dieta por ello te recomendaría:

A) Take a multivitamin.
B) Supplementation with Vitamin D, there are many formats, but the best known are capsules and drops.
C) Supplement of Zinc. the ones that I am consuming right now are these
D) Magnesium Supplement.

SIf you're going to buy the supplements yourself, read the labels to make sure you get a decent amount of the micronutrient.

Many people really underestimate nutrition, they think it's "posh," unnecessary, unimportant, etc., but remember that **if you want to have optimal levels of testosterone, it is not enough to just take enough micronutrients, sufiences proteins, etc., you have to take as much as possible** (without harming you because you are taking too much), if you want to do it only with food, would have to take 5 steaks, 7 salmon, 9 salads, 10 pieces of fruit, etc. per meal, this is just an example to give you an idea of what it would be like, if you did you would end up in the doctor in a short time, so you should consider taking supplements or multivitamins that are nothing more than condensed nutrients and put in a way that you are able to take.

32. Ashwaghanda will help you a lot.

What is Ashwaghanda?
It's an adaptogen that helps you increase testosterone levels.

How does he do it?
Ashwaghanda changes your testosterone levels at the brain level.

Ashwaghanda will also help to have lower cortisol levels in your blood, has anti-inflammatory properties, increases HDL and reduces LDL.

I personally recommend KSM-66 extract.

33. Probiotics.

Endocrine disruptors are seriously affecting our health, the endocrine system has glands that create and regulate hormones, the most important is testosterone, endocrine disruptors are substances that "deceive" the body by posing as hormones. This also happens with testosterone, as a result of which our body sometimes produces too many hormones or too few. The disruptors are found almost everywhere, everything you eat, touch, smell, etc is "infected" with disruptors: food, plastic bottles, air, sunscreen, etc.

Many studies have shown that probiotics help "fight" endocrine disruptors, mostly by excretion. In one study a group of rats exposed to bisphenol A (BPA) were given a probiotic. The results were as follows:

- The BPA in blood was much lower.
- There was much more bisphenol in the stool.
- The amount of BPA in urine and feces was more than 2 times higher in rats who took probiotics.

Therefore, according to this study, probiotics minimize the negative effects of bisphenol and help the excretion of this via urine and anal.
The best supplement is this, as it has all strains of bacteria belonging to the groups Bifidobacterium and / or Lactobacillus.

34. Less estrogen!!

The female hormone, estrogen, by degracia is not only present high in women, it is very common to find men with high levels of estrogen. This happens because testosterone is transformed into estrogen by the enzyme aromatase, the enzyme aromatase can be increased by: drinking too much alcohol, heating plastics in the microwave, being fat, drinking milk, using products with xanoestrogens, and so on. Apart from avoiding the habits mentioned above, there are also supplements that will help you remove the estrogen your body does not need. The best currently is **"Indol-3-Carbinol (IC3)"** which is present in vegetables such as broccoli, this compound makes it easier for the liver to eliminate estrogen when they are excessive.

35. The Tongkat Ali.

Do you want to stimulate the secretion of CYP17 enzymes in your testicles, would you like to suppress the hormone SHGB (sex hormone binding globulin), do you want to inhibit the enzyme aromatase to prevent your testosterone from turning into estrogen, the **Tongkat Ali** also called **Eurycoma Longifolia** can do this for you, of course this is scientifically proven.

36. Ginger increases testosterone.

Ginger increases testosterone by 17%, LH by 43% and FSH by 17% after 3 months of daily intake. It also has other anti-inflammatory properties. Normally ginger can be found in shops, supermarkets, etc, but if you live in a country where ginger is not very well known you can also find it in amazon.

37. Goat Grass In Heat.

This plant called **"goat herb in heat"** or epimedium contains icariin that elevates testosterone, as well as greatly improves the quality of erections, the "trick" is that the icariin is an inhibitor of natural Pde-5, most drugs to fight erections are inhibitors of Pde-5, no doubt if you have low levels of testosterone or problems with erections should take goat herb in heat or epimedium.

38. Mucuna Pruriens.

If you want to increase sperm volume and testosterone levels you should take **Mucuna Pruriens**.Scientists in one study gave 75 healthy men and 75 infertile men 5 grams of Mucuna for 3 months, in the end testosterone levels increased by 38% in infertile men and 27% in healthy men.They also increased luteinizing hormone.

Conclusion

Increasing testosterone takes work and is not easy (lifestyle, physical activity, diet, supplements, etc.), **be patient and see making changes gradually** to reach perfection and have optimal levels of testosterone.

Did you like the book?

CLICK HERE TO WRITE ME YOUR OPINION ON AMAZON

If you're not sure, send me a personal message.

BIBLIOGRAPHY

1- Sleep as much as you need.

1.1 Research.
1.2 Research.

2- Muscular mass and definition.

2.1 Research.
2.2 Research.
2.3 Research.
2.4 Research.

4- Endocrine disruptors and plastics are your enemies.

4.1 Research.
4.2 Research.
4.3 Research.
4.4 Research.
4.5 Research.
4.6 Research.
4.7 Research(BP-2).
4.8 Research(BP-3).

5- Sex is important.

5.1 Research(Strip Club).
5.2 Research.
5.3 Research.

6- Medications and their side effects.

6.1 Research(ISRS).
6.2 Research.
6.3 Research
6.4 Research(Sylfonylurea).
6.5 Research..
6.6 Research(Drug for hair lost).
6.7 Research(Spironolactone).
6.8 Research(ketoconazol).

7- The posture of your body.

7.1 Research.

8- The money.

8.1 Research (Brokers).
8.2 Research.
8.3 Research.
8.4 Research.

9- Your testicles.

9.1 Research.
9.2 Research.

11- Your Calorie Intake Matters.

11.1 Research.

14- Fats.

14.1 Research.
14.2 Research.
14.3 Research.
14.4 Research.

14.5 Research..

15- Veganism is mostly bad.

15.1 Research.
15.2 Research.

16. Ecological food.

16.1 Research.
16.2 Research.
16.3 Research..
16.4 Research..

17. Milk.

17.1 Research..

30. Never overtrain.

30.1 Research..

32. Ashwaghanda will help you a lot.

32.1 Research..

33. Probiotics.

33.1 Research..

35. The Tongkat Ali.

35.1 Research..

36. Ginger increases testosterone.

38. Mucuna Pruriens.

recipient reader. Under no circumstances will any legal responsibility or blame be held against the publisher or the author for any reparation, damages, or monetary loss due to the information herein, either directly or indirectly.

Respective authors own all copyrights not held by the publisher.

The information herein is offered for informational purposes solely, and is universal as so. The presentation of the information is without contract or any type of guarantee assurance.

The trademarks that are used are without any consent, and the publication of the trademark is without permission or backing by the trademark owner. All trademarks and brands within this book are for clarifying purposes only and are the owned by the owners themselves, not affiliated with this document.